Me, Again

How Postpartum Depression and Anxiety Transformed My Life

Bridget Croteau

Me, Again:
How Postpartum Depression and Anxiety
Transformed My Life

Printed in the United States of America
First Printing: 2018

ISBN-10: 0692199187
ISBN-13: 978-0692199183
Library of Congress Control Number: 2018911967

www.meagainbook.wixsite.com/home

Cover photo by Talia Salvador - Mix Photography
Back Cover Photo, Hair and Make-up by Beyond
Photography

To all my fellow "Warrior Moms"

You are *not* alone.

You are *not* to blame.

With help, you will be well.

You are loved.

You are beautiful.

You are incredible.

You are worthy.

You are amazing.

You are enough.

CONTENTS

PREFACE

Quite some time ago, I remember seeing a post on my Facebook feed about the Japanese art of Kintsugi. Kintsugi is the art of fixing pottery with lacquer and gold, silver, or platinum powder. According to Mymodernmet.com, instead of hiding the cracks and flaws or throwing out the item, it is repaired in a way that the repair is acknowledged, showing the history and "life" of the object. I thought it was truly beautiful, both in appearance and in practice.

As I thought about what I would write in this book. I couldn't help but think how Kintsugi was a great metaphor for my journey with perinatal mood and anxiety disorders, specifically Postpartum Depression and Postpartum Anxiety. I felt like the person I was before children was no longer there and altered in some way. However, through my journey of recovery, I was spiritually and mentally put back together and I am not exactly as I was before, but better, transformed, or more "beautiful" if you will.

And so, this is the general theme of this book - how postpartum depression and anxiety transformed me and what I learned.

INTRODUCTION

I am by no means an expert on PMADs or anything health related at all. I can only speak from experience and from what I have learned through educating myself. What I will say is that PMADs are *very* real and *very* common. This is not something made up, something to gain attention, or something to just "suck up."

Do not believe anyone who tells you otherwise.

Even though some celebrities (thank you to those who have been brave enough to share their story) have come forward to share their stories in the last few years and started conversations that are so overdue, there is still a stigma surrounding mental health in general, especially maternal mental health.

This is why I am writing this book. We need personal stories. We need to be able to connect to another mom and say, "Yes, I felt that too." We need to feel the hope that someone else went through this and is okay now, so I will feel better one day too. We need the assurance that this isn't our fault. We need to know that there are resources out there and people to reach out to.

Reading and hearing stories of survival from other women was a source of comfort to me while I was suffering with postpartum depression and anxiety. I desperately needed a connection and to feel like I wasn't alone. I hope this book serves the same comfort to you.

1

PLANS, PLANS, PLANS

I had *almost* always wanted to be a teacher.

There was a short time where I wanted to be a doctor

or geneticist, and also a period where I wanted to be

an author when I was in kindergarten (look at me

now; I was a smart kindergartener!). Soon after,

however, I fell in love with the sciences in middle

school and decided I would become a science teacher.

This part of my story may seem unrelated to my PPD/PPA journey, but I promise you it is! You see, in high school, I had high enough grades to be ranked among the top 10 students in my class. After earning a full scholarship, I set off to college to pursue my dream of becoming a science teacher. I loved my college (St. Joseph's) and the entire experience. Believing I would be an amazing and fun teacher, I had the lofty *and rookie* goals that my enthusiasm and love for learning would inspire a whole new generation of students.

I did well in college and was actively involved in the school community; I served as President, Vice-President, and Treasurer of the Biology Club over a three-year period, was a member of the Biology Honor Society, and participated in many school events.

After graduation, despite my grades, school involvement and references, I had a difficult time getting a job. I literally applied to every single science teacher position I was certified for from the Queens/ Nassau border to Montauk (and if you know anything about Long Island, that is quite the distance, filled with many school districts). I went on lots of interviews, but wasn't getting hired. The most common reason I heard was that they "really liked me" but hired the "other candidate" who had more experience.

How am I supposed to get experience if no one will hire me?

I was getting really discouraged but I kept interviewing until I finally landed a job a couple of weeks before the start of the school year. I knew I would love this job; it was perfect for me. I loved everyone who interviewed me and the position was for teaching middle school science (which is what I *really* wanted to teach!). I happily (and stressfully) taught at this position for four years until I was laid off because of budget cuts. I was granted tenure and excessed at the same time.

I was absolutely devastated.

I gave this job everything I had; I was an advisor for two after school clubs, volunteered for everything, and had excellent reviews. In my head I knew and understood that there was nothing I did or didn't do that caused this to happen, but I still felt awful. In fact, I felt like a failure, even though I put on a "happy" face for everyone. I didn't even tell my incredible students whom I had hoped I would be teaching again the following year.

To make matters worse, this school district, as well as many other school districts in Long Island, laid off many people that year. With so many teachers searching for a new job, there were very few job prospects. I was lucky to get a leave replacement job; unfortunately, I hated it. This wasn't the school district for me. I was miserable *all* year, and even had thoughts of quitting mid-year...but a quitter, I am not. I missed my previous school district and just wished they would hire me back.

The teaching job market was even worse during the next hiring season. Again, even though being laid off was fully out of my control, I felt like a complete failure. I didn't know what I was going to do career-wise with the rest of my life. Clearly, teaching again wasn't an option (at least for now). For the first time I felt like I lacked a direction. Should I go back to school and get another degree? I kind of liked the thought of going back to school, but had no clue what I should study.

I felt like I lost a big part of myself. Who was I if I wasn't a teacher?

I had naively filled my life with my career and didn't have hobbies or many friends outside of work. My life had revolved around my career and I tied a lot of my self-worth to my career accomplishments. Now what would I do? What was my identity? I felt like I barely knew who I was anymore.

If there is one thing my friends and family know about me, it's that I am a planner. I like order, I like structure, and I love goals. I always have schedules and plans for everything from the current day to five to 10 years in the future. I hated that I no longer had my "plan" and that the plan I had created and worked so hard to accomplish for years fell apart in front of me. What was I going to do without my plan? How could all this happen? I had a plan, people!

Since planning is my specialty, I also had a plan regarding having children. The "plan" originally included trying to get pregnant sometime in the 2011-2012 school year, since I would be tenured. We decided that if I was going to be unemployed, this was going to be the perfect time to have a baby. I mean, I was already home!

So while I was nearing the end of my year at the school district in which I felt miserable, I got pregnant with my first daughter.

And this is where my story begins....

2

THE ARRIVAL OF THE PRINCESS

I got pregnant with my first daughter during that not-so-wonderful teaching experience. We were elated and totally scared when we saw the two pink lines appear. This was real now, not just an idea. I now had a little baby growing in me.

My pregnancy was wonderful. I felt generally good, except for some lovely morning sickness. I craved orange Coolatta drinks from Dunkin' Donuts, wings, and french fries, and couldn't stand to eat eggs.

My doctor visits were pretty uneventful; the baby was growing well and I was doing just fine. I spent a lot of my free time reading books, blogs, message boards about what I should be prepared for in the coming months during my pregnancy, labor and beyond.

In one of the books, postpartum depression was discussed very briefly. This led me to do a little extra research on it too. I learned that because I had anxiety and depression in the past, I was at risk for postpartum depression and/or anxiety. I also learned that major life events, like losing a job, were also a risk factor.

In our minds, Beau and I thought we had prepared

ourselves by just basically "knowing" that postpartum

depression was a possibility. We really didn't know

what, if anything, we could do beyond understanding

this fact. So we didn't spend too much time thinking

about it after that - we just crossed our fingers and

hoped it wouldn't happen to me.

I wish there had been more information provided in

those books. Perhaps I would have prepared myself

more for the possibility of getting a perinatal mood or

anxiety disorder.

We spent the following months preparing for our little

girl's arrival - painting her room a sweet shade of

pink, decorating, and buying diapers, clothes, crib,

toys and other baby necessities. I cleaned the house

from top to bottom and cooked and froze meals to

have during those first days home. I did everything I could think of at the time to feel prepared for my baby's arrival (I told you I was a planner!).

We were ready. At night, while we watched our sitcoms and dramas, I bounced gently on our exercise ball (because I read it could help bring on labor), and hoped "tonight would be the night."

One day in early November 2011, I went to my weekly appointment with my nurse practitioner. All looked great...until I started to leak fluid. We were sent for a sonogram to make sure nothing was wrong. The sonogram technician said my daughter looked fine, but my amniotic fluid level was low. She left the room briefly to call our OB office and returned saying, "Congratulations, you're going to have your baby today! Your doctor wants you to go to the hospital for an induction."

I was not prepared for this.

I was *not* ready and this was *not* part of the plan.

I mustered a "thank you" and left the office in shock. We headed home to call our families, grab our bags, and have our labradoodle, Jake, picked up by our dog trainer and family friend.

We were scared. What was going to happen? What was an induction like? What would the doctor in the hospital say? Was I okay? Would the baby be okay? Why was my fluid low? How did this even happen? I was so careful! What did I do wrong?

A feeling of sadness came over me; I would never know what it felt like to count and time contractions while eating dinner or have my water break dramatically while happily shopping like it does in all the movies and on television.

We were admitted to the hospital and I was given Cervadil to get my body ready for the induction. The plan was to let the Cervadil work its magic for about 12 hours and then either do another round of it or start Pitocin, depending on how I responded to the medication. My parents came to keep us company and then went home with the plan of coming back in the morning. This was clearly going to take a while according to the doctor's plan.

Plans failed once again, however. After nine hours, nurses came running into my room, put an oxygen mask on me, and removed the Cervadil. I was so scared! What was going on?

I was told my baby's heart rate was slowing and I was in full-blown, painful labor. My contractions were long, painful, and happened one right after the other.

I was terrified.

I was in so much pain and begged for something to help me. Because I was so early in the labor I wasn't allowed to have an epidural yet and was given Demerol. The Demerol made me feel like I had one too many cocktails and I fell asleep for about an hour. I was woken up by even more painful contractions. Eventually, I was given an epidural and I felt much better!

The following day my parents, sister, her husband at that time, and my mother-in-law came to visit and anxiously awaited the arrival of our baby. Bless their hearts for waiting so long in the hospital with us - it took forever! It felt so great to have their company and with the relief the epidural provided, I brushed my messy ponytail and even put on some make-up while in bed. I wanted to look good in my first family photos. This made my family laugh and sort of roll their eyes.

After 30 or so hours of labor - including two hours of pushing - my precious little Natalie was born. Delivery took so long that the residents/interns who were in the room with my OB asked if they needed to intervene. My OB declined, saying while it was taking a long time, I was making progress. I kind of hated that the residents/interns spoke about me like I wasn't even in the room, but I was kind of busy, so I didn't give them a smart comment.

I had expected to feel beautiful waves of love when I held my little girl for the first time.

I didn't...*at all.*

Frankly, I was so exhausted, I wanted to pull all the wires and IVs off of me and just go to sleep. But I couldn't. During delivery, I spiked a low fever, and my daughter had a fever when she was born as well. She was taken from me after a quick cleanup and a couple of family pictures and brought to the NICU.

I was angry. I was scared. I was beyond exhausted.

After delivering my placenta, I was eventually taken to my room. My room was shared with another mom who had her baby rooming with us. My heart broke a little every time her baby cried. I begged the nurses to let me go see my baby. They refused. I argued again. I am not one to normally argue with authority, but there was no way they were keeping me from my baby girl.

If I could have felt my legs, I would have walked to the NICU myself (my legs were still numb from the epidural). They finally agreed and wheeled me down the hall to the NICU. My poor little baby was in an incubator covered in wires and monitors. My heart broke into a thousand pieces. I felt awful inside. I felt completely responsible for her being in there. If I had refused an induction would she have avoided this? Should I have not asked for an epidural? My baby is minutes old and I already felt like I was screwing up, that this was all my fault. I tried my hardest to fight back tears. I wanted her to be with me and I desperately wanted to feel the love and euphoric feeling I thought I was "supposed to" feel.

No one would let me breastfeed her at this time, and no one told me I should be pumping in the meantime. How was I supposed to know all of this? I don't even think I really knew what a pump was at this point. So I didn't, and I think this certainly played a role in my low milk supply that soon followed.

My daughter's NICU stay was very difficult. She remained there for a week before we were allowed to take her home. In the meantime, we struggled desperately to breastfeed her. We asked for help from anyone that could possibly help. She had so much trouble latching. My amazing husband went to multiple stores looking for nipple shields (who knew those were a thing) to help us on the recommendation of a NICU nurse.

I pumped and gave her formula to supplement. Because I was discharged before her, my husband and I took many trips a day to visit and feed her. Sometimes it would take us the better part of an hour to get her to latch, even with the nipple shield. Some nurses were amazing and so supportive and others were kind of annoyed that we were so insistent on breastfeeding. I do understand that their ultimate goal was to make sure she was fed and healthy enough to go home.

I desperately wanted to do something right by my daughter and have *something* go according to plan. I thought that if I could breastfeed her, it would

somehow make up for my "failure" with her birth and

NICU stay.

On the other hand, I also tried to tell myself that

Natalie was indeed the biggest and healthiest baby in

the NICU, so I should be happy. But I wasn't. There

were babies in the NICU with truly serious illnesses.

My baby just needed some observation and

antibiotics. This gave me an additional layer of guilt.

How dare I be upset when her story could be far

worse?

The day before Natalie was supposed to go home, a

nurse got a call from Infection Control and said I had

a candida infection on both sides of my placenta.

How scary does that sound? I pictured CDC

employees in HAZMAT suits coming to the NICU.

The nurse continued that Natalie's NICU stay would likely be extended. I broke down completely. I felt my insides just break into even more pieces than they already were. I couldn't move off the chair I sat on. I had tears just pouring down my face. I was failing. Again. My poor baby...stuck in the NICU because of me.

A pediatrician happened to be in the NICU when we got this news and he spoke to the nurses. After that conversation, he talked to us and told us it was okay. He looked at our records and the infection was so sparse. Natalie could go home the following day as planned and would be fine. I was so grateful for him talking to us. I really needed to hear that she was okay.

The next day, a week after she was born, we *finally* got

to take our little princess home. I couldn't wait to get

her home and to say goodbye to the incubator, wires,

monitors, IVs, and the hospital.

3

PPD, THE LIAR

Shortly after she came home, Thanksgiving and Christmas were around the corner. Holidays were kept low-key. I, sadly, don't remember a lot from those days. I do remember doing some online shopping (thank goodness for Amazon and Prime shipping), baking cookies, and decorating our Christmas tree with Natalie. I love the holidays and I was determined to make sure we had a calm and quiet but nice first Christmas.

It felt so good to bring our little girl home. Breastfeeding didn't get much easier; I still struggled greatly. In addition to breastfeeding, I pumped around the clock in an attempt to increase my milk supply. We also fed her formula. I kept record of the milliliters of milk I pumped. The constant pumping, cleaning, and breastfeeding became too much for me to handle, both time-wise and emotionally, but I just couldn't give it up. I was so desperate to feel like a "good" mom. In my head, I was already such a failure - this part of my plan *had* to work. If I couldn't make breastfeeding work, I would be a *total* failure. What had I done right up to this point? Absolutely nothing.

These thoughts consumed me.

Looking back, I don't know why I tortured myself like I did - and it was truly torture. My mind constantly told me how awful I was and that I was a failure. If I were to do it again now, I would never do this to myself. I would never encourage anyone I knew to do what I did. I hated pumping. I hated keeping record of my milk output. I hated researching better ways to breastfeed and how to increase my milk supply. I drank Mother's Milk tea, ate oatmeal everyday, and made "lactation" cookies. I knew formula was perfectly fine, but I had it set in my brain that "breast was best." I was determined to do the "best" for my baby. For those of you who may be struggling with this, *please* don't stress yourself out with feeding. Your sanity and health are important. Do what works for you, your baby, and your family. Remember, *fed is best* (even if it is through formula!).

I feel like I missed out on so much. Between the pumping and breastfeeding, cleaning pump parts, and researching, I don't remember a lot from my baby's first months. I can't tell you how old she was when she rolled or laughed for the first time or completed any of those early milestones. I was not very diligent with filling out her baby book either. I don't regret many things about my life but I do, to a degree, regret not enjoying these early moments.

I hate that my postpartum depression didn't allow me to enjoy this time. Postpartum depression is such an awful illness - it's a thief and a liar. PPD stole those precious early days with my daughter. These are moments I can never get back. This illness lied to me and truly made me believe that I was a horrible mom, wife, and person.

In the meantime, I put on a happy face for family and friends who visited. I would smile for pictures and answer their questions about being a new mom with the "right" and "expected" answers.

"Yes, I love being a mom."

"It's the best."

"I'm so happy."

I didn't feel this way *at all*.

If only people knew how often I cried. I wanted to scream.

"No! I hate being a mom."

"This was a mistake."

"I hate myself for feeling this way."

"Why am I so unhappy?"

"Please tell me I'm going to be okay."

"I want my life back."

"I want to run away. My husband and baby will be much better off without me."

I wanted to say all of these things to someone. Anyone. But I was so afraid of being judged. I didn't think anyone would understand. I just knew they would say things like, "but she's so cute," "she's such a good baby," "how could you be unhappy - you have a beautiful and healthy baby?" I knew people would say this, because I had these same thoughts. Natalie *was* such a good baby. A great baby actually. She was happy, absolutely beautiful, slept through the night at one-month old, and was clearly a bright baby. She loved to investigate and watch people and was curious about everything around her.

I knew what some of the signs of postpartum

depression were, but I honestly didn't think I had it. I

was in complete denial. I blamed all the bad feelings,

stress, and crying on being a new mom, the

breastfeeding issues, and the NICU stay. Who

wouldn't be stressed with a baby who was in the

hospital? Those rationalizations could make a little

sense for awhile, but months after she came home, the

NICU stay wasn't a good excuse for me feeling this

way anymore.

4

THE LIGHT AT THE END OF THE TUNNEL

The "light bulb" finally lit up in my brain when Natalie was approximately four months old. My husband was away on a bachelor party trip, leaving me home alone with the princess. I was okay for some of the weekend...but I then became really angry. I cried a lot. I was furious with my husband for being able to go away for a weekend.

I wanted a weekend away.

I hated that my life changed so dramatically and he could just carry on with his "normal" life. I became filled with emotions. I broke down and cried and let all of it out. I finally realized that I had been feeling all these emotions - anger, sadness, grief, loss, fear, confusion and anxiety - since my baby had been born. I wasn't myself and hadn't been in some time. I felt so alone; I felt like I didn't know who I was. Finally, through the tears, I had the thought: "Wow. I think I have postpartum depression."

Of course, I headed to Dr. Google. I began to read websites and reacquaint myself with the symptoms. One of the first webpages I read was titled, "The Symptoms of Postpartum Depression & Anxiety (in Plain Mama English)," on the Postpartum Progress website. As I read, tears streamed steadily down my cheeks. The way each symptom was explained hit me hard. They explained *exactly* how I felt. I didn't have *all* the symptoms, but I had some. I remember feeling relieved to see each symptom explained in an easy-to-understand and relatable way rather than clinical terminology.

I knew I had to tell Beau. I was scared what his reaction would be, but knew I couldn't keep this from him. He had a right to know and I would need his help and support to get through this. Once Beau arrived home, I turned to him and said, "I think I have postpartum depression." He didn't yell. He didn't say mean things. He didn't call me "crazy" or tell me to "suck it up." He simply said, "It's okay. We will find you help." I don't think he realized I necessarily had postpartum depression, but he knew something was off. I think me realizing this made him feel better too in some way.

The hospital sent us home with piles of flyers about various classes and baby information, and of course I saved them all. I found a flyer about a postpartum depression support group. That Monday I called the number and spoke to a wonderful woman who was in charge of perinatal education, including this group. She made me feel like it was going to be okay. Luckily, they had just started a session of the support group and I attended the following week.

I also reached out to my OB/GYN office. The receptionist scheduled me for an appointment later that week with the nurse practitioner. We saw her for most of our prenatal appointments. I really liked her; she made me feel comfortable. When I saw her for this appointment she was sweet, caring, and understanding. I could tell she really felt awful about the way I was feeling and wished she could do something about it. She told me that this wasn't my fault. She gave me a list of resources to call for therapy. Unfortunately, the numbers were out of service, no one answered, or they weren't working, which really disappointed me.

One thing that was successful was the support group. I cannot say enough good things about this group. I finally felt like I wasn't alone! Everyone there had a different story, but we shared many similar thoughts and feelings. I didn't speak often, but I did share my story, feelings, and concerns. I felt at ease and at home in this group. I looked forward to each meeting. Each week had a theme and the facilitators stressed for us to take care of ourselves. One of the analogies they made often was that of oxygen masks on an airplane - you are told to put *yours* on first before helping others. If you aren't okay, you won't be able to help anyone else.

With the exception of attending the support group and therapy, I hadn't been caring for myself like I should have for quite some time. My husband had been encouraging me for years, even before having our baby or being pregnant, to find a hobby and do something I enjoy. I never made finding a hobby or having fun a priority. Honestly, I didn't even know what I would enjoy doing. I was always "too busy" with graduate school, teaching, lesson planning, and after school clubs to find the time for fun. I also couldn't justify the financial cost to myself. I still struggled with the idea of making time for myself, but eventually came around and started ballroom dance

lessons when Natalie was just over one year-old
(which I still do and absolutely love).

I continued attending the support group and was so
grateful for the encouragement and information it was
pouring into my life. One amazing feature of this
group was "Family Night." At this meeting, moms
were invited to bring their family members and
support system (spouse, siblings, parents, close
friends, etc.) so they could learn more about perinatal
mood and anxiety disorders. At the meeting we met a
mom, Wendy, who was now a volunteer with the
Postpartum Resource Center of New York. She wrote
her own book about her experience with postpartum
depression and postpartum OCD (her book is
excellent, by the way). We also met her mother, who
had also become very involved in volunteering for this
cause. We were able to hear their story from both

perspectives - as a mom who went through it and from someone who cared for her during that time.

My parents, my husband, and our baby attended the "Family Night" meeting with me and we were all incredibly grateful for this experience. Everyone appreciated hearing both women's perspectives and learning more about their experiences. My mom, much like me, wanted to learn more. She purchased each of us a copy of Wendy's book and asked several questions, including how she can help me.

After this meeting, I felt a glimmer of hope!
Maybe I would feel better one day too.
Maybe I could volunteer for this cause when I am better!

I knew I had a long way to go, but this was one of the first little specks of light at the end of the tunnel I saw. I felt truly thankful to hear her story and see that she was doing better. In fact, she was actually more than okay; she was sharing her story at events and helping so many other moms.

5

FAKE IT UNTIL YOU MAKE IT

I attended every meeting in this session of the support group. The women in my group were amazing, as were my facilitators. Still in contact with several of my fellow group members, I'm incredibly thankful to everyone I met through this experience. Their advice was greatly appreciated and knowing that we supported each other was an added bonus

Everyone knew my issues with breastfeeding. With the help of my group mates, facilitators, and from my family, I slowly weaned Natalie. We stopped breastfeeding completely by the time she was seven-months old. It was emotionally hard to wean her, but it was also such a relief. I felt a boulder of pressure slowly fall off my shoulders.

Even though it was difficult, I knew that it was the best for both of us to wean. It wasn't healthy for me to be so stressed and depressed. She would be just fine without "mommy milk." By this point, she was eating some solid foods and honestly, didn't care whether her milk was from her mom's breast or was formula in a bottle. She just wanted to eat!

In addition to the support group, I also attended therapy. For a short period of time I actually saw two therapists. One therapist specialized in perinatal mood and anxiety disorders and the other was a general therapist. After speaking to me and giving me two tests, a therapist diagnosed me with postpartum depression and postpartum anxiety, with the depression being the "bigger" of the two issues at the time.

Both therapists were wonderful and I very much appreciated that I could go to therapy with my baby in tow. It was such a relief to not have to search for childcare!

I very slowly started feeling better. I always describe my recovery as more of a roller coaster rather than an incline. I would have several good days and then a bad day, followed by a few good days and a couple more bad days. But generally I trended (slowly)

towards more "good" days than bad.

I credit a lot of my recovery to the work I did. I

expressed my honest feelings and worked through

them in therapy and my support group. I also read

books by moms who went through postpartum

depression (you'll find my favorites at the end of this

book). I tried my very best to dig myself out of the

hole I felt I was in. I desperately wanted to feel better.

I knew enough to know that recovery wasn't going to

just happen on its own - it would take effort, work,

and time.

There were many days I didn't want to do anything. I

forced myself to get out of bed, to take the princess to

library classes, play with her, read to her, and cuddle

her. I desperately wanted that connection that we

were *supposed* to have. I would plaster on my "happy face" for the public, put on clothing that wasn't sweats, and apply make-up. Make-up always made me feel like a woman and a human again. It still does; I rarely leave the house without *at least* concealer and mascara! I figured I would "fake it until I make it."

I felt like I couldn't let other people know I was such a mess inside. I still didn't think many people would understand what I was going through. I feared their judgment. I tried my best to look the part and like "I had it all together."

Please don't think that everyone else *is* okay because they *look* okay. I am "Exhibit A" to show the mask we sometimes put on to hide the way we really feel. Part of me wishes I didn't put on a mask all the time. I wish I could have been more transparent and open to those in my life who didn't already know what was going on.

Despite my best efforts, I also had many feelings and thoughts of just wanting to run away. I swore that my husband and baby would be fine or even better than fine without me. My husband, mom, and dad would often remind me that this was a ridiculous thought. Clearly my daughter loved me very much and she would obviously be far better off having me in her life.

When Natalie's first birthday approached, I had a decline in my mental health. I began reliving her birth, her NICU stay, and all the feelings I had following this. I couldn't make birthday plans without the old feelings and memories coming back again. I cried frequently. One day I broke down and I told my husband I couldn't have a second baby and that I didn't want any more children. I just couldn't do all of this again and couldn't understand why anyone would risk living through this more than once. I don't think he ever took those statements too seriously because he knew I was suffering at the time.

After her first birthday, I couldn't take it anymore. I hated that I had made so much progress only to see all my work and efforts plummet with my declining mood. I made an appointment with my primary care doctor and a psychiatrist. I wanted to see if I needed medication or if something else was "off" biologically.

My primary doctor ran a whole gamut of blood tests. She found that my B_{12} was on the lower side of normal and actually fell into a range where increased levels of depression were found. My doctor told me to take B_{12} vitamins daily (I still do), but warned me it would take probably a month or so to feel any better if this was truly the issue.

My psychiatrist appointment wasn't until I was on B_{12} for nearly a month. The psychiatrist I spoke to didn't think I needed any medication. She thought I could work though this and be okay. But she wrote me a prescription anyway. I never filled the prescription because the B_{12} was helping me.

Shortly after seeing the psychiatrist, I started ballroom dance lessons. I had wanted to try this type of dancing since my time in graduate school. I never made the time, had difficulty finding classes, and could never rationalize the cost (ballroom lessons are not cheap!). Beau had encouraged me to find a hobby and was thrilled that I picked something to try. He didn't even mind the cost because he was so happy I was doing something for myself.

I immediately fell in love with these dance lessons. I felt free, at ease, and at home. I could laugh. My dance lessons helped me tap into a side of me I didn't know I had. I could be creative and expressive, sassy and fun, or sexy and fierce. I was able to play with my personality. I gained confidence. I finally had time with other adults!

Over the years, I have even done three showcase dance routines - swing, tango and rumba – in front of actual people! I will never consider myself overly talented at this hobby, but I really do love and enjoy it, even though it isn't easy. My instructor, John, has become a part of my family. I know I can always talk to him and he can always cheer me up.

I highly recommend making the time to do something for yourself, whether you are struggling from postpartum depression or not. I am so glad my support group stressed this point to us many, many times. Caring for yourself doesn't have to be expensive or time consuming. It can be as simple as a walk around the block or taking a shower alone; it's really whatever *you* need in that moment.

6

PREGNANCY #2

When Natalie was about 18 months old, my husband and I decided to try for baby number two. We were blessed and thrilled to become pregnant that month. I not-so-secretly hoped for another girl. I wanted Natalie to have a sister and a best friend. My wish came true! Our families were so excited to add another member to the family.

Shortly before becoming pregnant, I switched from my prior OB/GYN to a midwife group associated with a large local hospital. I had heard wonderful things about this practice and hospital from several friends. I was excited to work with them and appreciated their gentler, less invasive approach and was hopeful my birth experience would be different this time. As a bonus, I heard the rooms were private; no more sharing with another mom! Yes!

This pregnancy was pretty good. I definitely suffered from more morning sickness. I never went *anywhere* without saltine crackers, Chex, or Cheerios cereal in my purse. I continued with therapy while I was pregnant. I did struggle with some feelings of guilt and anxiety.

I felt guilty bringing another baby into the world when I felt my first daughter didn't get the "best of me" when she was a baby. I didn't know how she would react to having a new sister or brother and I definitely didn't want her to feel like I was replacing her.

I was anxious about what my mental health would be after I had the baby. I worried about caring for a toddler and a newborn. How was I going to manage two children? Natalie was now entering her "terrible twos." How could I manage that *and* a newborn while running on probably little to no sleep?

I worried about what the baby's birth would be like. I prayed the birth wouldn't be as awful as the last and prayed there would be no NICU this time. I talked about all these feelings and thoughts with my therapist and my family. Everyone assured me that everything would be okay and that many of these feelings were very common and normal.

I made sure I talked to my midwives as well. The midwives were made fully aware of my history of postpartum depression, my birth experience, and breastfeeding issues with my first daughter. They appreciated how open I was about my experience. All of the midwives I encountered were incredibly caring and nurturing. They often asked me how I was feeling during my prenatal visits and truly seemed interested in my feelings and concerns.

Much like we did for her sister, we searched for names, painted her room a lovely shade of light purple, prepared her room with an adorable theme, filled her closets and drawers with diapers, wipes, and clothes (many were her sister's old clothes - a definite perk to having two girls born close together). I

cleaned the house from top to bottom; I even

vacuumed the floor in our unfinished basement! And,

I once again prepared a freezer full of meals for when

she was born. We also tried to prepare our oldest

daughter for the new baby. We purchased books for

her about being a big sister and had a gift "from the

baby" ready for her when the baby arrived - a teddy

bear and a baby doll of her own to care for.

That fall, my mother-in-law was diagnosed with lung

cancer. She had surgery a couple of months later to

remove the tumor. Surgery went well, but the doctors

wanted to do chemotherapy in January to help make

sure this cancer wouldn't return. Her first

chemotherapy appointment was around when the

baby was due to be born. We knew my mother-in-law

would have her own health to care for, so we looked

into other options of extra help for when the baby was born. We were definitely nervous about having less "hands on deck," especially with my history. But, we were also very concerned about my mother-in-law's health and wanted her to do whatever was necessary to become healthy again.

One of the support group facilitators told me about postpartum doulas. I had *no* idea what that was! I heard of birth doulas, but never a postpartum one. I was quite intrigued and researched it that very week. My husband and I found an amazing doula that was knowledgeable in postpartum depression, anxiety, and other PMADs. She was also a lactation consultant. Her fees were completely reasonable as well. We were sold!

My husband planned on being home for three weeks after the baby was born. We hired our doula to come when he returned to work and to be with us until the baby was three months old. We planned on her coming three days a week for three hours a day to help me with whatever I needed at the time.

7

CROTEAU, FAMILY OF FOUR

I went into labor on a snowy night in late January (of course, a January labor story in New York wouldn't be complete without snow). I had painful contractions that came at short, regular intervals. I called my mom to come over to watch Natalie. I also called the midwives to let them know what was happening. While we waited for my mom, I packed my final items and took a warm shower to help with the contractions (by the way, it didn't help!). Once my mom arrived, she took one look at me and said, "Go! Now!" She could tell by my face that it wasn't a good idea to wait at home at all. I was having lots of contractions very close to each other. I wasn't expecting to have to leave so quickly.

The hospital is about 40 minutes away and it was snowing. Luckily, the roads weren't completely awful yet and were totally empty because it was *very* early in the morning. We were lucky to follow behind a snowplow for part of our journey. My contractions were so painful, I was *almost* convinced that my baby would be born on the side of the road in my car. My husband did an amazing job navigating the snow in a safe but efficient manner and keeping me calm while listening to me moan and scream with my contractions.

I was already somewhere between seven to eight centimeters dilated by the time we arrived. The midwives took such great care of me and encouraged me. I begged for an epidural, the midwives obliged, even though they assured me that I could absolutely finish labor without one - especially since I was almost done. The epidural didn't work on me this time and I felt *everything*.

I should have taken the midwives advice. After a grand total of six hours of labor (a breeze compared to the first labor), my second little girl, Chloe, was born that snowy January morning. She was beautiful and much bigger than her sister - two full pounds heavier to be exact.

She also had quite the set of lungs! She cried for two whole hours *non-stop* after she was born - no exaggeration. No matter what we tried, she just wouldn't stop. Nurses would leave the room, return fifteen minutes later, look at us and ask, "Is she still crying from before?" We would just look back at them and nod. I thought, "Oh my goodness, am I in for a ride with this kid; she's going to be a tough cookie." I sure was right; she is stubborn, willful, and still likes to cry (she's four now). Chloe is also hysterical, sweet, loves to cuddle, very smart, and *adores* her sister.

Throughout the day, she only wanted to be held. Anytime I put her down she would return to crying (no naps for mommy). We had trouble breastfeeding again as she wouldn't latch well. "Oh, here we go again," I thought. Chloe also had instances of rapid breathing. One of the nursing assistants was quite worried about it and scared us. She kept coming in my room to check on our vitals and insisted that Chloe needed to go to the nursery and see a doctor immediately because her breathing was abnormal.

I completely broke down. I watched through the nursery window while doctors and nurses checked her. The sight of her being surrounded by several medical professionals scared me and brought back memories of her sister's hospital stay. I sobbed into my husband's chest and clung to his shirt. "This can't be happening again," I moaned through the bawling.

Shortly after that, the doctor came out and said Chloe was totally fine. He explained that newborns breathe like this sometimes. I was so relieved. I appreciated the nursing assistant's concern, but in the moment, I wanted to yell at her for putting us through that ordeal unnecessarily. I knew there was no way for her to understand our past experiences and how sensitive and scared I would feel about this, but the situation made me a little angry.

The next day my husband went home to shower, check on Natalie, and show off pictures of her little sister. My dad came to visit me and baby Chloe in the hospital. I loved seeing him and he was so excited to meet the baby. He updated me on how Natalie was at home and I told him all about the birth and how Chloe likes to cry.

Later that day, we all went home! I was so happy to be released from the hospital, return to my other baby girl, and have Chloe meet my mom, Natalie, and our fur-baby, Jake.

8

EARLY DAYS HOME

I was thrilled to be home. I was exhausted, of course, but I actually felt pretty good. I was so excited that we were able to go home early and only spend one night in the hospital. This hospital was fantastic and the food was pretty good, but nothing beats home sweet home!

I wasn't crying all the time like I did with Natalie. Chloe quickly learned to breastfeed like a champ and with a little help from my mom and a visit from my doula/lactation consultant, we were doing great.

We did have a hard time with helping Natalie adjust to being a big sister and not being the only child. She loved her sister and loved being included in the care of her sister. Natalie would bring me diapers, help put dishtowels away, and help load the laundry in the dryer. But, she began acting out towards us, especially Beau. She screamed, threw tantrums, hit, and even bit him. I felt so bad for Beau. He was trying so hard to help everyone. It broke my heart to see Natalie take her feelings out on him.

We did discipline her, generally a time out or loss of a toy, but also made an effort to make sure we spent extra special time together. We enjoyed painting,

baking, reading, or cuddling with just the two of us (or

just Natalie and her dad). We knew that Natalie was

still little herself and this was a huge adjustment for

her. I never wanted her to feel like we didn't have

time for her anymore or that she was being replaced.

She loved the one-on-one time, and I did too. My

parents also spent special time with her when they

would come to visit.

My parents were amazing and incredibly helpful when

we returned home. In the weeks that followed, they

visited often and *never* came without meals in hand

for us (thank you mom and dad!). My mom was

insistent on helping with laundry and other

housework. Like any Italian mom (or really, any

mom) she made it her mission to make sure that I ate

enough. She prepared yummy and huge lunches for me and made sure I kept up with my water intake.

When Beau returned to work, our amazing doula came to help me three days a week for a few hours. Having her with me was simply amazing. I took naps, ran errands alone, took the kids to doctor appointments without having to bring both with me, and could take a moment to relax. She vacuumed. She played with the kids. She helped me with breastfeeding, pumping, and getting Chloe to take milk from other people. I wanted to be able to be away from her for more than two hours. Her presence was so comforting. I knew I would be okay *because* she was there. I am so thankful for her help; she was simply amazing. If you have a baby on the way, I highly recommend looking into postpartum doulas!

Chloe was not an easy baby. Almost every day around dinnertime she cried for at least an hour. Non-stop. We tried everything. We fed her, rocked her, burped her, did bicycle movements with her legs, tried to distract her, lights on, lights off, tried to put her down to sleep, put her in bouncy chair, her swing, laid her tummy down on her play mat, laid her back down - you name it, we tried it. Nothing ever helped.

I struggled with the crying. While the cry-fest went on, I was a mess. I didn't know what else to try and felt just horrible about myself. I hated her cries. The crying made me feel anxious and angry every day this happened. Sometimes I cried along too. I would call my mom on the phone and cry. The cherry on top was that our labradoodle, Jake, cried every time one of my girls cried (and he still does). My house felt like a zoo!

I couldn't imagine why this little baby just cried all the time.

We, of course, told her doctors about the excessive, almost daily crying. She had no signs of reflux, but her doctors thought that it was possible she had silent reflux and gave us a prescription for a generic antacid. They told us that if she does have reflux it will help, if not, then it won't. But in the meantime, it wouldn't harm her either way. We began giving it to her as prescribed. I can't say for sure if it helped, but *eventually* she stopped crying like this when she passed the three-months-old mark. We were so thankful that it had stopped. It was really trying our patience and I don't know if I could have managed it for much longer. We kept her on this medication until she was over a year old.

9

THE "C" WORD

My mother-in-law had her first chemotherapy
appointment right before Chloe was born. She did not
feel great after her treatment (who does?), but she was
able to mostly bounce back within a week or so.

A few weeks later she had her next treatment. This
time she did not bounce back so well. She had a very
hard time staying hydrated, became very weak, and

needed an IV of fluid to rehydrate. Beau was called to her house several times that week to help with her care. I tried to help how I could. I made her some of her favorite meals in an attempt to help her eat something and called to check on her often.

Everyone was deeply worried about her. I worried for her health and for my husband's well being. Neither of us were sleeping well; he was working full-time, trying to help me with our infant and two-year old, and worrying about and caring for his sick mom. It was a stressful time.

The next treatment she had totally knocked her off her feet. She was very sick. She was brought to the hospital and we found out she needed surgery. Following the surgery, she remained in the hospital for almost a month. She was so weak, that after the hospital stay she was sent to a rehabilitation facility to gain strength back before going home. We were scared that we would lose her. She almost died.

My poor husband was extremely stressed. I encouraged him to seek therapy and find ways to relieve his stress, including playing soccer, going for jogs, or using the treadmill or elliptical. He took my advice and went to therapy for a few months; unfortunately, I don't think it helped him much. I don't think he was as open to the process as he could have been and I don't believe this therapist and Beau were a great match. Sadly, finding a therapist that took evening appointments was not an easy task. As I'm sure any of you who have tried to contact a therapist know, several don't return phone calls, aren't taking new patients, or only have open appointment times that are impossible for your schedule.

Fortunately, today, my mother-in-law is doing well. She recovered her strength, gained back her weight, and is back to her normal self.

10

HELLO, ANXIETY

When Chloe was three months old, my doula left. After her departure my mental health began to slowly decline. Chloe was not sleeping well at night and was still feeding every two to three hours around the clock. I was exhausted. I was stressed and worried about my husband and mother-in-law. I was trying to raise a wonderful, but jealous two-year-old and an infant. It was a lot to deal with, and eventually I couldn't deal with it all.

By the end of May, Chloe had numerous bad nights where she would be up for most of the night. She wasn't always crying, just awake. I couldn't sleep if she was awake. I remember one particular night when she was still in the basinet in our room. We tried everything - feeding her, burping, putting her in a rock n'play, music on, music off - you name it. I broke down in tears and just sobbed. I'm pretty sure my husband did too. I was so tired. I was so frustrated. I just needed rest. My body, mind, and soul were tired.

After those hard nights, we talked to her doctor and she had suggested moving her to her own space. Moving Chloe to her own room would allow us to get more rest and she might be more comfortable there.

We put sheets on her crib mattress. With her doctor's

blessing, we added a small stuffed animal in a corner

of her crib where she couldn't really reach to give her

some sort of comfort and company. Let me add, she is

still very attached to this stuffed animal to this day. It

is a small pink elephant; she calls it "Pink Mama."

One of her first words was "mama" and of course, I

thought she was talking to me. Nope. It was her

elephant "mama." Thanks, Chloe!

During this time I was convinced that Chloe hated me.

I told my mom and husband on several occasions that

Chloe just didn't like me and that is why she wouldn't

sleep. She was trying to drive me crazy. I knew this

was silly, but I really just didn't feel like she loved me.

I was so exhausted that I couldn't comprehend her

love for me at this point. I felt like she only wanted me there to feed her every two to three hours.

Chloe definitely slept better in the crib in her own room than in her basinet in our room. She still woke up multiple times per night to feed, which is "normal" from my understanding for breastfeeding babies. Her doctors and nurses swore she should be sleeping in longer stretches then three hours, and any breastfeeding moms and resources I talked to swore it was normal and totally fine for the multiple night waking periods at this point in development. I didn't know who to believe, all I knew was that I was extremely tired.

I had a very difficult time getting back to sleep post-feeding, especially the last one, which was around three or four o'clock in the morning. Her feeding would last for 15 or so minutes, but I typically remained awake for an hour or so past the feeding time. This remained the norm for months. I was so tired. The exhaustion made me become really anxious about many things, but mostly about Chloe and her sleep schedule.

I began to obsess about what time she went down for naps, the length of time between naps, and making sure she was down for her nap at a specific time. I began to follow the "90 Minute Sleep Program." It worked beautifully with regards to getting Chloe to nap and catching her sleep cues. However, it drove me into a very anxious and schedule obsessed mode. We couldn't leave the house if it was close to her naptime. Ten minutes before naptime I would start soothing her with sounds, like a hair dryer or rain falling, and rocking her.

I could feel the anxiety building inside of me when she refused to fall asleep. There were many times I felt like I would explode. The thoughts in my head would race: "If she doesn't sleep now, she will miss X minutes of nap. She won't sleep tonight. Not sleeping tonight will put her into a sleep deprivation and she will never sleep again. Then I will never sleep again." These thoughts would repeat over and over in my head and I would burst into tears and cry. My thoughts snowballed so much that I went from a missed nap to never, ever sleeping ever again.

At the time these thoughts made complete sense to me, but now they are clearly not very rational (and I consider myself to be a pretty rational and logical person). To me, that is one of the awful things about PMADs — they make you think and feel things that aren't true. These disorders "take over" some of your thoughts and feelings, taking the "rational you" and turning her into "irrational you."

I also began feeling incredibly angry when the anxiety would build up inside me. I yelled often. I punched and kicked walls and I threw things. This behavior is *very* uncharacteristic for me. I hated feeling like this. I didn't like screaming or acting like I did in front of the kids. I would try to scream or throw something in another room, but I know I did this in front of them plenty of times. I lost some self-control. I am not proud of this at all. I would feel bad afterwards and tried to make sure I apologized to my kids when I calmed down.

Because of what I went through before, I realized I needed to talk to someone. I knew that I was suffering from anxiety, even if I didn't realize that all my thoughts were from anxiety. I called therapists who had afternoon appointments available, and my amazing mom could come and watch the girls after work. Thank you, Mommy!

My therapist wasn't specifically trained in PMADs, but was aware of what they were and understood. I do, however, highly recommend seeking someone who is educated and trained in PMAD. My therapist was caring, loving, and made me feel safe in her space and was always available for me to text or call if necessary. In fact, my husband did call her one day during an argument we were having while I was having a panic attack about schedules, leaving the house, and missing nap times. She was really helpful in calming me down and also talking to my husband to help him understand what I was going through.

11

MY FRIEND FERBER

Therapy helped me with strategies to not lose my cool as often in front of the girls and to calm the anxiety attacks. I did deep breathing, put Chloe in her crib (even if she cried), and gave myself a few minutes to calm down. I let myself cry and hit a pillow and do what I needed in that moment.

Of course it didn't always work.

trying a sleep training method that did not

ive letting the baby cry. Chloe cried enough as it

as - I didn't want to hear more! It worked to a

degree. She did learn to soothe herself more than

before, but still couldn't seem to master doing it in the

middle of the night. I believe we were doing two

middle of the night feedings at this point. When she

cried, I would wake up, feed her, and put her back to

bed.

Some of the strategies we followed were: putting her

to bed sleepy, but not asleep, having a routine (which

we already followed), and encouraged her to use a

pacifier or suck her thumb (neither which she liked as

a baby).

To help myself get back to sleep when I finished

feeding Chloe, I began drinking lavender tea at

bedtime and using lavender essential oil in a diffuser in my room. It did help to calm me and get me to sleep quicker. But I unfortunately still had issues going back to sleep after her feeding in the early morning.

Eventually the exhaustion just made my mind so irrational that I was truly convinced that there was something physically wrong with Chloe. This had to be why she just couldn't sleep all night. I used "Dr. Google" to read about babies who don't sleep well and tried to find out what was wrong with her.

I also took her to see her pediatrician and explained how she just doesn't sleep. I told her that Chloe still needs to be fed in the middle of the night even though she was seven months old. I said there has to be something wrong. What could it be? A sleep disorder? A vitamin or nutritional imbalance? Or just something biologically "wrong"?

I'll never forget what her doctor said next: "Your baby is just fine. We will run some blood work to make sure, but who I am really worried about is *you*." She went on to strongly suggest sleep training with the Ferber method and explained what it was. She also asked about me being in therapy or a support group (my children's doctors knew I had PPD before) and wanted me to make sure I took care of myself.

We left the office and took Chloe to get her blood work done. I called my mom on the way and told her what Chloe's pediatrician said. She agreed with the doctor and also strongly encouraged me to try the Ferber method. Bless my mom, because she was also so concerned for my health, she offered to sleep train

Chloe for me! I was convinced that this method wouldn't work and was just going to make me feel awful. But, I reluctantly agreed, mostly so I could say, "I told you so!" My mom started sleep training that same day.

In case you didn't guess already, Chloe's blood work was fine.

Beau, my mom, and I read the relevant chapters in the Ferber method book. My mom offered to do the first two days of sleep training and Beau and I would do day three. We put the girls to bed as normal and then Beau and I slept in our downstairs living room and let my mom work her amazing magic.

The first night, there were lots of tears. It was hard to listen to as we could still hear everything even though we were on a different floor. But, it was a relief to not be the one dealing with the tears. I remained awake and was very tense the entire time she cried. Beau held me and stroked my arms and hair to calm me down. He reassured me that it would be okay.

My mom swore to me, that even though there were so many tears, Chloe was trying so hard to soothe herself and was doing so great at it. Night number two was easier than the first. Chloe was learning quickly to put herself back to sleep and learning that she wasn't being left alone or being ignored - mommy and daddy were nearby. Night three was scary for me, but wasn't that bad at all. Chloe even woke up happy and smiling! Her smiling at me in the morning made me smile. This meant the world to me. I had felt so guilty and anxious about sleep training her, but she was totally fine.

As the days went on I began to feel more rested and energized. My anxiety was far from gone, but because I wasn't as exhausted, I was better able to handle these feelings and not lose my cool as quickly. I continued to go to therapy, my support group, and my dance lessons. Everyday, I felt a little more like "me" and even felt some hope and excitement for my future.

12

GLITTER, GLAM AND FINDING ME

A little known fact about me, in fact no one knew this until recently, I have wanted to compete in pageants since I was a teenager. I was afraid to ask my parents to let me compete in one because I was fearful they wouldn't allow it (I still don't know why this made me afraid). I also knew pageants could be very expensive.

As a teenager, I suffered from low self-esteem and had depression as well. I always wanted to be perfect and anything short of perfection made me feel worthless. I never felt pretty either. I knew if I competed in a pageant, I would surely lose (and probably be in very last place), and so, I never expressed this desire to anyone and never competed.

I let fear stop me from doing something I felt I wanted to do.

As I grew up, I was so busy with college classes, schoolwork, clubs, and jobs that I never pursued it as a young adult either. The next time I even thought about pageants was when I started feeling better after my postpartum anxiety with Chloe.

I randomly heard about Mrs. Pageants and was intrigued. *Maybe* this was my chance to compete! I thought this could be a great opportunity for me. It would allow me to get involved in my community and maybe even do something to help moms who had postpartum depression or anxiety. I also thought it could be an opportunity to make new friends, have some fun, and have something to focus my energy on (besides my children, of course!).

I began doing some research and was amazed to find many "Mrs." pageants. The searching was a little overwhelming as there were so many choices. I found the Mrs. New York America pageant website and thought this pageant sounded amazing. I emailed the director, Diane, and heard back from her quickly. We had a phone conversation shortly after that. I loved her from that first conversation...and still do!

I felt like I *needed* to compete in *this* pageant. There were only a couple of months to prepare for the 2014 pageant. I knew I was nowhere ready to compete, so I didn't. But, I did sign up for the following year and competed in my very first pageant in November 2015 as Mrs. Suffolk County America. I spent that year volunteering, learning about pageants, learning to walk in six-inch heels, finally taking care of my health through exercise (which I used to hate, but have since grown to love), and cleaning up my diet.

I had an amazing time competing, even though I had no idea what I was doing and was utterly terrified while on stage! My husband, kids, and my parents came to watch and cheer me on. Everyone was so proud of me, even though my husband said I looked like a "deer in headlights" on stage (I really did though; He wasn't lying). They were proud of me for using this experience to share my story, raise awareness, and for stepping so far out of my comfort zone. It takes a lot of guts to get on stage - especially in a bathing suit - and to put yourself out there in that way.

I felt a calling to return to this pageant and so I competed again in 2016, 2018, and I will be competing once again in March 2019. My platform continues to be, "You Are Not Alone: Raising Awareness for Perinatal Mood and Anxiety Disorders." I continued working with the Postpartum Resource Center of New York and became more and more involved each year. Pageants or not, I will always remain involved in this amazing organization.

My experience with the Mrs. New York America pageant has helped me find and use my passion to raise awareness and educate people about PMADs. It gave me that extra push and courage to step way out of my comfort zone and speak at events, meetings, trainings, and to our local news channel and media outlets about my personal story. I know the sash gives me a larger and louder microphone and platform in which to share my story, and I want to impact as many people as I can. I feel a deep need to use my voice to help moms, dads, and families who are going through what I went through.

I am forever grateful to the Mrs. New York America pageant, including my amazing director, the pageant staff, and my fellow contestants. Never in a million years would I have expected to grow as a person and learn as much about myself through this pageantry journey as I have. This experience has most certainly played a role in allowing me to "put myself back together" (along with therapy, support group meetings, and dance of course).

13

LESSONS LEARNED

My experiences with postpartum depression and postpartum anxiety were truly the most awful times of my life. While I would never wish this on anyone, I am oddly grateful for the experience. I know that must sound very strange, but this experience gifted me with so many lessons.

Probably the most important lesson that I learned was that it is okay to ask for help. I feel like, we as women, put this unnecessary pressure on ourselves to "do it all." I always had a bit of an issue asking for help. I always felt I needed to do things myself, especially relating to my personal life. I think I felt pride in being able to do and take care of things on my own and also a shame or embarrassment for asking for help in the first place.

As a stay-at-home mom these feelings were multiplied for me. I was home with my daughters all day. I always thought I should be able to do all the things they need. But the reality is, even though I am home with them, I still need help. Sometimes I just need a break.

Taking care of myself is important too.

I cannot care for my family if I am an empty mess and have nothing left to give. I am lucky that I have family

I can call on for help and a babysitter that my girls just absolutely adore. Had I not gone through PPD and PPA, I don't think I would have ever learned to ask for help and to accept the help people offer to me.

I had depression and anxiety previously in life; I always was really hard on myself. I put pressure on myself to be perfect and I never really felt pretty. I think I always was looking for approval and acceptance as a teen and young adult. I still don't really understand why. But what I do know is that overcoming PPD and PPA was hard and when I got through it, I grew to be really proud of myself. It wasn't easy, but I did it!

This awful and difficult experience made me realize that I had so much more strength, passion and fire inside of me than I ever knew I had. After I felt better, I *knew* I had to share my story. I felt a calling inside to do so. The newly found qualities gave me the courage to try new things and step *way* out of my comfort zone to begin competing in pageants and using my pageant title to help share my story. The title of Mrs. Suffolk County America has opened so many incredible doors to me; speaking to various audiences, including nursing leadership, support group facilitators and attendees, creating and co-teaching a webinar, and speaking to local media. The pre-PPD me would have been far too scared and fearful of other's judgment to even dream of participating in any of these activities.

When I felt depressed not only did I feel alone in the sense that no one else would understand, but also felt just truly alone. Motherhood, in general, can be very isolating. I learned that I wasn't alone. Through my support group and book reading, I found a community of moms who "got it."

They totally understood the struggle with depression and anxiety.

They understood the guilt.

They understood the shame.

They understood the loneliness.

I learned that you are truly never alone. No matter what you are experiencing, there is someone else out there who understands what you are feeling and is going through a similar situation.

Being able to share my story and help other moms, dads, and families has been incredibly healing to myself as well. It has been difficult to write this book. There were lots of tears while writing. There were times I had to stop and begin writing again another day. But it feels so good to have this out there on paper. Books written by other moms helped me a lot, and I hope that my story helps you too.

14

A LITTLE ABOUT PMAD

PMAD stands for perinatal mood and anxiety disorders, which according to PostpartumNY.org, is a "general term used to describe a wide range of emotional disorders a woman can experience during pregnancy and after the birth of her child."

There are many mood and anxiety disorders that fall under the PMAD umbrella including depression, anxiety, PTSD (post-traumatic stress disorder), OCD (obsessive compulsive disorder), bipolar disorder, and psychosis. These can happen at any time during pregnancy or in the first year following the birth of the baby.

PMAD can happen to anyone (it occurs in 1 in 5 mothers), but there are risk factors that put certain individuals at higher risk than others. Just like any other medical condition, having risk factors doesn't mean you will have a PMAD because you are more at risk, and just because you do not have any risk factors doesn't mean you will not get a PMAD. I think it is very important to be educated about PMAD either way.

Dads can be affected by this as well (it is estimated to occur in 1 out of 10 men). Some risk factors include (but are not limited to): previous trauma, personal or family history of depression or other mood/anxiety disorder, lack of support, unplanned pregnancy, major life change, child in the NICU, and difficult pregnancy.

Postpartum depression/depression during pregnancy is very common among pregnant moms and postpartum moms. Some symptoms include (but are not limited to): crying, feelings of guilt, insomnia or sleeping too much, feeling inadequate, hopeless, worthless or overwhelmed, feeling irritable, having trouble bonding with your baby, and appetite changes.

Postpartum anxiety is also very common. Symptoms include (but are not limited to): anxiety, panic attacks, racing thoughts, trouble sleeping, feelings of dread, appetite changes, and feeling worried.

Postpartum obsessive compulsive disorder occurs in approximately nine percent of postpartum mothers. According to the book *Beyond the Blues*, some symptoms include repetitive behaviors, repetitive and/or intrusive and persistent thoughts, and feeling awful about the intrusive thoughts.

This book also shares that post-traumatic stress disorder occurs in approximately "six percent of women; rates are higher (up to 30 percent) in parents who have a child in the intensive care unit." Symptoms can include recurrent nightmares, extreme anxiety, and reliving of past traumatic events. Some risk factors include traumatic birth, previous traumatic events, and a baby in the NICU.

Bipolar disorder has two types: Bipolar I and Bipolar II. The risk factors are having a personal or family history of bipolar disorder. Symptoms include depression, racing thoughts, trouble concentrating, little need for sleep, and continuous high energy.

Postpartum psychosis is very rare - occurring in 1 to 2 out of 1000 women - but it is a medical emergency. Immediate help is needed in this situation. Symptoms include confusion, delusions, hallucinations, mania, and paranoia. These symptoms may come and go.

To learn more about PMADs, I highly suggest reading *Beyond the Blues* by Dr. Shoshana S. Bennett and Dr. Pec Indman. This is an excellent read and includes information about PMAD, a chapter for mother's going through a PMAD, a chapter for partners, one for siblings/family/friends, medical professionals, treatments, and a list of resources.

Treatment for PMAD may include any combination of social support (like a support group), therapy, or medication. It is also highly suggested that you see your primary care doctor for a complete physical. Be sure to take care of yourself; eat, drink plenty of water, exercise, and get rest (I know this is easier said than done sometimes, but it is so important).

PMADs cannot really be prevented (even some celebrities with *all* the resources one could have have suffered from them), but there are things you can do to make your life a little easier.

Prepare yourself; gather therapist names, find support group information, hire a doula, and gather your team of people to help you. Have these names and contact information ready and set aside in case you need it. Decide who you will call if you are in need (your choices could include your OB, a midwife, your therapist, or a primary care physician).

Next, stock that freezer! When you get home after having a baby, the last thing you're going to want to do is cook. But you do need to eat. Freezing easy meals to throw into a Crockpot or meals that are easy to defrost (lasagna/baked ziti/soups/chili) make your life a lot easier; it's one less thing to have to do or decide on.

Decide who will be your support at home. This support can come from: a spouse, parent, in-law, sibling, neighbor, friend, doula, extended family, babysitter, co-workers, or a member of your faith organization. Think about who can you talk to without fear of judgment or if you know someone who went through this before.

If you are a family member or friend of a pregnant or postpartum mom (or a new/expecting dad), please ask them how *they* are doing. I know everyone wants to see the baby, but it's not *all* about the baby. Listen to their answer. Please don't judge them as new parents judge and question themselves enough already. Let the new mom/dad tell you their feelings and concerns. Offer any help that you can give. This could range from letting mom nap, take a shower, run an errand, or get a manicure while you watch the baby.

Consider bringing over a meal, doing a load of laundry, and loading or emptying the dishwasher. If she (or he) is struggling, reassure them that this is not their fault and that they will be okay with help. If they don't have resources available, help them find some. Offer to call their insurance company or search their provider database. Offer to search for or make calls about support groups. Your support will mean a lot to them, even if they don't express it right away. I know that they will be grateful and appreciative of your help and support. Remember to also take care of yourself, especially if you begin to spend a lot of time caring for a struggling mom and/or dad. PMADs can affect everyone in the family, so it is important to take care of yourself as well.

SELF CARE IDEAS

Self-care is a relatively new concept to me. I didn't quite understand what this was before I had PPD. It can honestly be so many things, but simply put, it is anything that *you* need in that moment. The following are just some ideas rather than an exhaustive list. Also, keep in mind that self-care doesn't have to be expensive (although some choices can be):

- Take a bubble bath
- Go to coffee/dinner/drinks with a friend
- Take a walk around the block or further (alone or with baby in stroller)
- Workout (yoga, running, walking, weight lifting, hiking, etc.)

- Get a pedicure, manicure, massage, facial, or other spa treatment
- Run errands *alone* while someone babysits
- Read a book *alone*
- Watch a guilty pleasure television show or movie
- Say "no" to an activity or event you really don't want to go to; remember, you *do not* have to say "yes" to everything!
- Spend a day in your pajamas and relax and cuddle with baby
- Go to therapy or a support group
- Chat with a friend or family member
- Have some ice cream (or your favorite treat) and watch one of your favorite movies
- Take a class or lesson (perhaps a paint night, craft or dance class) that you enjoy
- Revisit goals and aspirations you had prior to having children

- Write or draw in your journal

- Take a nap

- Have a dance party with your child(ren) or alone

- Draw or color (coloring has been found to help reduce anxiety)

PERINATAL MOOD AND ANXIETY DISORDER RESOURCES

You are not alone. You are not to blame. With help,

you will be well.

New York State

Postpartum Resource Center of New York

www.postpartumny.org

Long Island Doula Association

www.lidoulas.com

Worldwide

National Suicide Hotline

www.suicidepreventionlifeline.org

1-800-273-8255

Postpartum Support International

www.postpartum.net

2020 Mom

www.2020mom.org

Jenny's Light

www.jennyslight.org

The Bloom Foundation

www.thebloomfoundation.org

DONA International

www.dona.org

<u>**Blogs and Websites**</u>

Postpartum Progress Blog

www.postpartumprogress.com

Symptoms of Postpartum Depression &

Anxiety (in Plain Mama English)

www.postpartumprogress.com/the-symptoms-of-

postpartum-depression-anxiety-in-plain-mama-

english

Postpartum Dads

www.postpartumdads.org

RECOMMENDED BOOKS

Bennett, S. S., & Indman, P. (2010). *Beyond the blues: Understanding and treating prenatal and postpartum depression & anxiety.* California: Moodswings Press.

Edwards, L. (2016). *A dark secret.* CreateSpace Independent Publishing Platform.

Isnardi, Wendy. (2011) *Nobody told me: My battle with postpartum depression & obsessive-compulsive disorder.* New York: Legwork Team Pub.

Kleiman, K. R., & Raskin, V. D. (2013). *This isn't what I expected: Overcoming postpartum depression.* Boston, MA: Da Capo Lifelong, a member of the Perseus Books Group.

Kleiman, K. (2005). *What Am I Thinking?: Having a baby after postpartum depression.* Xlibris Corporation.

Kleiman, K. (2016). *Moods in motion: A coloring and healing book for postpartum moms. CreateSpace Independent Publishing Platform.*

O'Keeffe, G. (2008). *The Stork's revenge: My struggles and triumphs over postpartum depression. Deadwood, Oregon: Wyatt-MacKenzie Publishing, Inc.*

Shields, Brooke. (2006). *Down came the rain: My journey through postpartum depression.* New York: Hachette Books.

WORKS CITED

Bennett, S. S., & Indman, P. (2010). *Beyond the blues: Understanding and treating prenatal and postpartum depression & anxiety*. California: Moodswings Press.

My Modern Met Team. (2017, October 03). Kintsugi: The Centuries-Old Art of Repairing Broken Pottery with Gold. Retrieved January 3, 2018, from https://mymodernmet.com/kintsugi-kintsukuroi/

Postpartum Resource Center of New York. Learning About Perinatal Mood and Anxiety Disorder including Postpartum Depression. Retrieved April 19, 2018, from https://postpartumny.org/ppdpmad/

ACKNOWLEDGMENTS

Words cannot express my gratitude to my family and friends for their support and love through both experiences with perinatal mood and anxiety disorders and through the experience of writing this book. This has been a labor of love and I am so grateful for your help, support, and encouragement.

Thank you to my husband, Beau, for being not only a wonderful husband, but being my best friend. I don't know what I would do without you. You have truly been my rock when I needed you most. Thank you for always supporting my dreams. I love you!

To my mom and dad, Marguerite and Frank, thank you for all you have always done for me; I wouldn't be who I am today without you. Thank you for encouraging me to write this story and always being my biggest cheerleaders and supporters. Thank you for *always* being there when I needed you. I am a very, very lucky girl to have parents like you.

To my beautiful daughters, Natalie and Chloe, mommy loves you more than words can say. Thank you for being your unique, beautiful, wonderful selves and for teaching me so many amazing lessons. I love you to outer space and back.

To my mother-in-law, Geraldine, I know we didn't talk much about what was going on during this season, but I truly and deeply appreciate that you were always there when I needed help and never asked for or needed a reason why. Your support allowed me to start taking care of myself and allowed me to heal.

To Sonia, thank you for being such an amazing and inspiring woman. The Postpartum Resource Center of New York has helped countless moms, dads, and families, including mine. I am forever grateful to you! Thank you for your friendship and for always believing in me.

To Wendy, thank you for all the work you have done (and continue to do) including writing your book and speaking at the Circle of Hope support group's Family Night back in 2012. You are amazing, and that night was one of the first times I felt any significant hope about *my* future. I cannot thank you enough for that precious gift of hope. Your story inspired me to continue working to get better and to give back when I was "me" again.

To Karen, thank you for being an amazing facilitator and running the Circle of Hope support group. This group was the biggest piece to my recovery. Thank you for creating this space where I felt safe and cared for, and where I could share my feelings and experiences without any judgment.

To Kate, you are amazing. I am so thankful that we found you! I can never thank you enough for taking care of my girls and me after I had Chloe. Your presence in my home helped me to feel like everything would be okay and it was calming to all of us. Everyone looked forward to the days you were here; Natalie enjoyed your visits just as much as I did.

To John, I don't think I ever expressed to you just how much my ballroom lessons with you mean to me and how they have been an important piece in my recovery from postpartum depression and anxiety. Thank you for always being so understanding, kind, and making me be able to laugh, especially on the days I had a hard time finding anything to smile about. I can always count on my lesson with you to cheer me up and to brighten my day.

ABOUT THE AUTHOR

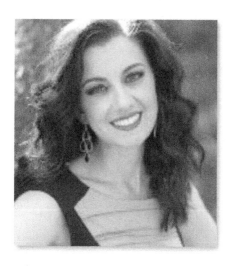

Bridget Croteau lives in Suffolk County, New York, with her husband, Beau, their two children, Natalie and Chloe, and labradoodle, Jake. After her experience with PPD and PPA, she has been an active volunteer with the Postpartum Resource Center of New York, sharing her story in order to help moms, dads, and families. She is currently serving as Mrs. Suffolk County America 2018-2019 to help bring awareness to this important cause.

Hair, Make-up and Photograph by Beyond Photography

Made in the USA
Middletown, DE
11 January 2019